KNOWLEDGE GUIDE TO
OSTEOMYELITIS

Essential Manual To Diagnosis, Treatment, Prevention, and Advanced Therapies for Bone Infection Management

DR. AARON BRANUM

Copyright © 2024 BY DR. AARON BRANUM

All rights reserved. Except for brief quotations embodied in critical reviews and certain other noncommercial uses permitted by copyright law, no part of this publication may be reproduced, distributed, or transmitted in any form or by any means, Including photocopying, recording, or other electronic or mechanical methods, without the prior written permission of the publisher.

Disclaimer:

The data in this book, is solely meant to be informative and instructional.

This book is not intended to replace expert medical advice, diagnosis, or care. No medical, health, or other professional services are offered by the author, publisher, or any affiliated parties

Individual outcomes may differ in the practice of these therapies, which entail a variety of approaches and methodologies.

A one-on-one session with a trained or certified healthcare professional is still preferable. It is best to consult a trained healthcare provider before making any decisions regarding your health.

The author of this book is not affiliated with any specific website, product, or organization related to any of these therapies.

All reasonable measures have been taken by the author and publisher to guarantee the authenticity and dependability of the material contained in this book

Contents

CHAPTER ONE 13
  BONES' ANATOMY AND PHYSIOLOGY 13
    Bone Structure 13
    Bone Remodeling And Development 14
    Blood Flow To The Bones 15
    The Function Of The Bone Marrow 15
    The Value Of Strong Bones......................16

CHAPTER TWO 19
  THE MORPHO PATHOLOGY OF OSTEOMYELITIS 19
    How Bone Infections Are Acquired 19
    Mechanisms Of Infection In Bones...........20
    Antibody Reaction To Osteomyelitis 21
    Osteomyelitis: Acute versus Chronic 22
    Problems Associated With Infection Of The Bone 23

CHAPTER THREE 25
  ASSESSMENT OF OSTEOMYELITIS............25
    Clinical Assessment 25
    Imaging Methods 26

Lab Examinations...................................27
Distinctive Diagnosis 28
The Value Of A Correct Diagnosis 29
CHAPTER FOUR..31
TREATMENT OPTIONS...............................31
Antibiotic Treatment............................31
Procedure 33
CHAPTER FIVE 37
STRATEGIES FOR PREVENTION...................37
Appropriate Wound Care: 37
Controlling Risk Factors: 38
Recommendations For Vaccination: 39
Prophylactic Antibiotics: 41
Importance Of Patient Education:............42
CHAPTER SIX...45
DIFFICULTIES AND RISK AREAS................45
Risk Factors For Osteomyelitis Development
....45
Possible Difficulties................................47
Effects On Mobility And Everyday Life 49
Techniques To Reduce Difficulties............51

    The Value Of Frequently Following Up 53
CHAPTER SEVEN 57
    ORTHOPAEDIC OSTEOMYELIA 57
        Particular Difficulties In Pediatric Cases 57
        Children's Diagnosis And Treatment Considerations 58
        Effects Of Psychology On Families And Children 61
        Prevention Techniques Particular To Pediatrics 62
CHAPTER EIGHT 65
    MANAGING OSTEOMYELITIS 65
        Changes In Lifestyle 65
        Exercises For Rehabilitation 67
        Coping Mechanisms And Emotional Assistance 69
        Extended-Term Management Strategies ... 70
        Keeping An Eye Out For Recurrence 71
CHAPTER NINE 73
    SCIENCE AND UPCOMING VIEWS 73
        Current Research Trends In Osteomyelitis 73

Treatment Strategies That Look Good 74
Obstacles In Prevention And Treatment 76
The Value Of Multidisciplinary Cooperation 78
Promoting And Endorsing Osteomyelitis Research 79

CONCERNING THIS BOOK

"Knowledge Guide to Osteomyelitis" provides a thorough exploration of the complexities of this crippling illness, serving as a beacon of knowledge in the field of bone health. Its core focus is on the anatomy and physiology of bones, including their formation, structure, and the vital function of bone marrow.

The book highlights the importance of bone health by establishing this fundamental knowledge, paving the way for a thorough investigation of the pathophysiology of osteomyelitis.

The pathophysiological pathways of osteomyelitis are precisely examined within its pages. The hazardous path that pathogens take to infect bones, the immune response's heroic resistance, and the striking differences between acute and chronic symptoms are all explained to readers. The book painstakingly describes the diagnostic journey as the story progresses, stressing the critical role of clinical evaluation, cutting-edge imaging methods, and the significance of a precise diagnosis in determining the best course of therapy.

When it comes to therapy, the book acts as a compass, pointing doctors toward a wide range of therapeutic alternatives.

Every option is carefully investigated, from the tried-and-true toolbox of antibiotic therapy to the complexities of surgical intervention and cutting-edge medicines.

However, the book goes beyond treating osteomyelitis; it also addresses prevention, promoting immunization, appropriate wound care, and patient education as the first lines of defense against the disease's never-ending assault.

Furthermore, "Knowledge Guide to Osteomyelitis" offers support to individuals coping with the consequences of this illness. Through the implementation of lifestyle modifications, emotional support, and long-term management strategies, it provides persons navigating the complex maze of osteomyelitis with comfort and empowerment.

The book's focus on pediatric problems, which recognizes the particular difficulties that children and their families encounter and provides specialized advice and support, is another example of its all-encompassing methodology.

The book goes beyond its immediate focus and into the fields of advocacy and research, illuminating emerging patterns, promising therapeutic modalities, and the critical necessity of multidisciplinary cooperation.

As evidence of its steadfast dedication, "Knowledge Guide to Osteomyelitis" advocates for increased awareness, support, and progress in the field of osteomyelitis research in addition to acting as a compilation of knowledge.

CHAPTER ONE

BONES' ANATOMY AND PHYSIOLOGY

Bone Structure

The body's amazing structures, bones provide for movement, protection, and support. They are made of a variety of tissues, including marrow, blood vessels, cartilage, bone, and nerves.

An osteon, the fundamental building block of bone, is made up of concentric layers of bone matrix encircling a central canal that houses nerves and blood vessels. Bones are made strong and flexible by this arrangement.

Cortical or compact bone, the outermost layer of bone, is robust and dense, offering support and defense.

The trabecular, or spongy, bone sits underneath the cortical bone. It is less dense and more porous, allowing gaps in the bone marrow and promoting the flow of waste materials and nutrients.

Bone Remodeling And Development

Ossification, a process that starts in the embryo and involves the progressive replacement of cartilage by bone tissue, is how bones form.

Bones continue to expand in length and width during childhood and adolescence until they achieve maturity.

The continuous process of remodeling involves the steady breakdown and replacement of old bone tissue with new bone. Whereas osteoclasts are in charge of bone resorption, osteoblasts are in charge of bone creation.

Because of their ability to repair micro damage and adjust to variations in mechanical stress, bones are kept strong and healthy by this dynamic equilibrium.

Blood Flow To The Bones

Bone health and function depend heavily on blood flow. Numerous arteries supply blood to bones; these vessels pierce the outer cortical bone and branch out into smaller vessels that are distributed throughout the bone tissue. These blood arteries help with bone formation, repair, and maintenance by supplying the bone cells with oxygen, nutrients, and immune cells.

The Function Of The Bone Marrow

The soft, gelatinous tissue called bone marrow is located inside the hollow cavities of bones. There are two varieties: red marrow and yellow marrow. Hematopoiesis, the process by which red marrow makes red blood cells, white blood cells, and platelets, is what gives blood its color. The majority of the cells in yellow marrow are fat, and they store energy.

A vital component of the immune system, bone marrow not only produces blood cells but also acts as a storehouse for immune cells, bolstering the body's fight against illnesses and infections.

The Value Of Strong Bones

For general health and well-being, maintaining bone health is crucial. Strong bones support the body structurally, safeguard important organs, and promote mobility. Numerous issues, such as osteoporosis, osteomyelitis, and fractures, can be brought on by poor bone health.

Eating a balanced diet full of calcium, vitamin D, and other minerals necessary for bone formation and maintenance is critical for promoting bone health. Frequent weight-bearing exercises, like jogging, strength training, and walking, serve to strengthen and promote bone remodeling. Maintaining bone density and preventing bone loss can also be achieved by abstaining from tobacco and heavy alcohol use.

People can help maintain their bone health and lower their risk of developing illnesses related to bones by learning about the anatomy and physiology of bones and implementing healthy lifestyle practices. To maintain ideal bone health throughout life, routine check-ups with medical specialists can also aid in the early detection and treatment of any underlying bone disorders.

CHAPTER TWO

THE MORPHO PATHOLOGY OF OSTEOMYELITIS

How Bone Infections Are Acquired

When bacteria or other pathogens enter the bone, osteomyelitis results. These infections usually enter the bone through many routes. Hematogenous spread, or dissemination through the bloodstream, is one frequent method.

This process involves bacteria infecting the bone by moving from another diseased place in the body, like a skin wound or lung infection, and settling there through the bloodstream.

Direct vaccination is another method by which diseases get into bones. This may occur as a consequence of trauma, such as a fracture or an open incision that exposes the bone to germs, or it may occur after surgery. Furthermore, infections from neighboring soft tissues, such as muscles or tendons, can travel to the bone. This is particularly true when the soft tissue infection is left untreated or inadequately controlled.

Mechanisms Of Infection In Bones

When viruses get to the bone, they can stick to its surface and begin to multiply, which can result in infection. The tough surface of the bone creates the perfect conditions for bacteria to grow and create biofilms, which are bacterial populations shielded by a slimy matrix. This makes it more difficult for the illness to spread and for the immune system and medications to work.

Bacteria can cause damage to blood vessels within the bone in addition to directly invading it, which would impair the bone's blood supply. This further weakens the bone's resistance to infection by impairing its ability to absorb vital nutrients and oxygen.

Antibody Reaction To Osteomyelitis

The immune system of the body is essential to the body's response to osteomyelitis. The immune system reacts to bacteria invasion of the bone by seeing them as foreign intruders and starting an inflammatory process. To neutralize the pathogens, immune cells such as white blood cells are brought to the infection site as part of this response.

On the other hand, immunological dysregulation in chronic osteomyelitis may result in tissue damage and prolonged inflammation. Without focused therapy, this may lead to an infection and inflammatory cycle that is hard to escape.

Osteomyelitis: Acute versus Chronic

Depending on the length and intensity of the infection, osteomyelitis can be categorized as acute or chronic.

The symptoms of acute osteomyelitis usually appear quickly and include severe inflammation, fever, and localized discomfort. Acute osteomyelitis is frequently curable with medications and surgery to remove diseased tissue if it is detected and treated quickly.

On the other hand, chronic osteomyelitis takes longer to manifest and is frequently linked to recurring or persistent infections.

Untreated acute infections can lead to chronic osteomyelitis, as can underlying medical problems that compromise the immune system's capacity to combat infections.

A combination of medications, surgical debridement, and, in certain situations, bone grafting to encourage healing is frequently needed for the treatment of persistent osteomyelitis.

Problems Associated With Infection Of The Bone

Several consequences, such as joint degeneration, systemic infection, and bone necrosis, can result from poorly managed or untreated osteomyelitis.

Bone necrosis is the result of an infection that kills bone tissue, resulting in the sequestrum—dead or devitalized bone—forming.

This may weaken the bone's structural integrity and raise the possibility of fractures.

If the infection moves from the bone to adjacent joints, inflaming them and harming the surrounding tissues and cartilage, joint degeneration may result.

In the afflicted joint, this may lead to persistent discomfort, stiffness, and loss of movement.

When osteomyelitis is severe, it can result in a systemic infection, which is a bloodstream infection that spreads to other parts of the body and can cause septic shock or sepsis.

A systemic infection is a potentially fatal illness that needs to be treated aggressively with antibiotics and supportive care as soon as possible.

CHAPTER THREE

ASSESSMENT OF OSTEOMYELITIS

Clinical Assessment

A vital first step in diagnosing osteomyelitis is a clinical assessment. It entails a comprehensive evaluation of the patient's past medical history and present symptoms.

Medical practitioners check for symptoms like warmth, redness, swelling, and localized pain in the affected area.

In addition, they record any recent surgeries or injuries that would have increased the patient's risk of developing bone infections. They also assess the patient's general health as well as any underlying illnesses like diabetes or immunodeficiency diseases that may exacerbate osteomyelitis.

Clinicians obtain vital information through this thorough assessment that directs additional diagnostic procedures.

Imaging Methods

Because imaging techniques provide detailed representations of the diseased bone and surrounding tissues, they are essential in the diagnosis of osteomyelitis.

Because they are easily accessible and can identify anomalies in the bone, X-rays are frequently the first imaging modality to be employed.

They can show telltale symptoms of osteomyelitis, including swelling of the soft tissues, periosteal response, and bone loss. However, X-rays could miss early-stage or subtle alterations, which means more sophisticated imaging modalities are needed.

When it comes to identifying osteomyelitis early on and evaluating soft tissue involvement, MRI (Magnetic Resonance Imaging) is very helpful because it provides better soft tissue resolution than X-rays. It has a high degree of sensitivity in detecting bone marrow edema, abscess formation, and tissue inflammation. Computed tomography (CT) scans are helpful for assessing bone morphology and offer comprehensive cross-sectional images of bone structures, particularly when surgical intervention is being considered.

Lab Examinations

In order to establish the diagnosis of osteomyelitis and determine the causative organism, laboratory tests are used in addition to clinical and imaging data. Blood cultures are frequently carried out in order to identify bacterial infections that are present in the blood and help choose the best medications. The process of collecting bone tissue samples for microbiological and histological study is known as a bone biopsy, and it is widely regarded as the gold standard for diagnosing osteomyelitis. This makes it possible to evaluate the integrity of the bone tissue and identify the infectious agent directly.

Distinctive Diagnosis

It's critical to distinguish osteomyelitis from other musculoskeletal disorders in order to avoid misdiagnosis and guarantee timely treatment. Differential diagnosis is crucial since conditions like cellulitis, septic arthritis, and neoplastic bone lesions can have similar symptoms. To rule out other diagnoses and confirm osteomyelitis, medical experts take into account a patient's clinical presentation, imaging findings, and laboratory data.

The Value Of A Correct Diagnosis

When osteomyelitis is diagnosed accurately, prompt and efficient treatment can be started, reducing complications and improving patient outcomes. Misdiagnosis or delayed diagnosis can cause the infection to worsen, destroy bone, and spread bacteria throughout the body, which raises the risk of morbidity and death. In addition, a precise diagnosis aids in the selection of the most effective antimicrobial medication, which helps to eliminate the pathogen and lower the risk of repeated infections. By highlighting the significance of a precise diagnosis, medical professionals prioritize patient safety and provide the best possible treatment for osteomyelitis.

CHAPTER FOUR

TREATMENT OPTIONS

Antibiotic Treatment

The mainstay of the osteomyelitis treatment regimen is antibiotic therapy, which attempts to eradicate the infectious agents that are causing the inflammation of the bones.

The microorganism under suspicion, the extent of the illness, and any underlying medical conditions of the patient all have a role in the selection of antibiotics.

To successfully treat the illness and stop its recurrence, a combination of antibiotics may be recommended in several instances.

Antibiotic delivery routes can change based on the type and severity of the infection. Oral antibiotics might be adequate in minor cases or as a post-treatment measure after intravenous therapy. However, antibiotics are given intravenously to ensure quick and direct distribution into the bloodstream, maximizing their potency, for more serious illnesses or when intravenous access is required.

Another important factor to consider is the length of antibiotic medication. Treatment regimens usually last for a few weeks to months, during which time medical professionals closely monitor the patient's progress and make necessary adjustments. Even if symptoms subside, patients must follow the prescribed antibiotic prescription religiously in order to stop the spread of antibiotic resistance and the recurrence of infection.

Notwithstanding the efficaciousness of antibiotic therapy, various obstacles can surface, including the emergence of drug-resistant bacterial strains or unfavorable drug responses. To get the best results in these situations, medical professionals might need to reevaluate the treatment strategy and look into adjunct therapies or other antibiotic alternatives.

Procedure

Surgical surgery is essential for the treatment of osteomyelitis, especially when antibiotic therapy is not effective or when complications like necrotic tissue or abscess formation occur. Removing the contaminated tissue, accelerating wound healing, and preserving the structural integrity of the damaged bone are the main goals of surgical intervention.

A fundamental component of surgical intervention, demineralization techniques entail the surgical excision of necrotic or infected tissue from the afflicted bone and its surrounding tissues. Careful debridement not only removes the infection source but also fosters an environment that is favorable to tissue repair and antibiotic uptake, increasing the effectiveness of later therapeutic approaches.

When an infection or surgical debridement results in bony flaws or voids, bone grafting may be necessary to fill them. In order to support bone regeneration and structural stability, bone grafts might be made of synthetic materials, donated bone, or the patient's own bone (autograft). This supplemental treatment helps to lessen the chance of fracture or deformity while also helping to restore the integrity of the damaged bone.

Furthermore, new treatment approaches and tactics to enhance patient outcomes and quality of life are being offered by continuing research and developing medicines, which have the potential to advance the field of osteomyelitis care.

These could include immunomodulatory treatments, targeted drug delivery methods, and regenerative medicine strategies meant to improve tissue regeneration and fight antibiotic resistance.

Future discoveries that shed light on the complex mechanisms underlying osteomyelitis could lead to ground-breaking approaches that completely alter the way the disease is treated.

CHAPTER FIVE

STRATEGIES FOR PREVENTION

Appropriate Wound Care:

One of the cornerstones of preventing osteomyelitis is making sure that wounds are properly cared for, especially in those with open wounds or injuries. Whether the wound is a small cut or a surgical incision, it is important to keep it clean and free from contaminants. This is routinely washing with a light soap and water, then putting on a sterile dressing and an antiseptic solution. It is imperative to keep an eye out for any indications of infection, like elevated redness, swelling, temperature, or discharge from the incision. Osteomyelitis can be averted by paying quick attention to any changes.

Furthermore, because they are more likely to develop foot ulcers, which can act as entry points for germs that cause osteomyelitis, people with diseases like diabetes or peripheral vascular disease need to take particular care when it comes to foot care. Osteomyelitis can be prevented in large part by practicing good foot cleanliness, wearing proper footwear, and regularly inspecting the feet.

Controlling Risk Factors:

One of the most important ways to prevent osteomyelitis is to recognize and control risk factors. A person's risk of getting this bone infection may be increased by specific medical conditions and lifestyle choices. For example, immunodeficiency diseases, diabetes mellitus, peripheral vascular disease, and malnutrition are all recognized risk factors. The chance of having osteomyelitis can be considerably influenza, for instance, are advised, especially for those who are more vulnerable, such as the elderly, small children, and people with specific medical conditions.

Osteomyelitis and other secondary consequences are less likely when the incidence of these infections is decreased.

Healthcare professionals need to be up to date on the most recent immunization recommendations from reliable organizations like the World Health Organization (WHO) and the Centers for Disease Control and Prevention (CDC).

Promoting the necessary immunizations among patients, particularly those who are more vulnerable, can have a major impact on overall infection prevention methods, which include osteomyelitis prevention.

decreased by addressing these underlying disorders with appropriate medical care, lifestyle changes, and nutritional support.

Apart from physical ailments, certain lifestyle choices like smoking can also hinder the healing of wounds and raise the chance of infection.

As a result, those who smoke should have access to counseling and programs for quitting, as doing so can both improve general health and reduce the risk of complications like osteomyelitis.

Recommendations For Vaccination:

Immunization is a potent strategy in the fight against several illnesses that might cause osteomyelitis.

Vaccinations against Haemophilus influenzae type b (Hib), pneumococcal bacteria, and

Prophylactic Antibiotics:

To stop osteomyelitis from developing, prophylactic antibiotics may be used in some high-risk circumstances. This prophylactic measure is frequently used in patients with weakened immune systems or in situations where there is a high danger of infection, such as prior to certain bone or joint surgery procedures.

Numerous variables, such as the type of operation, the medical history of the patient, and regional patterns of antibiotic resistance, will influence the choice of antibiotic and length of prophylactic treatment. To prevent antibiotic resistance, healthcare practitioners must carefully consider the advantages and disadvantages of using antibiotics prophylactically and follow evidence-based recommendations.

Importance Of Patient Education:

Empowering patients with knowledge about osteomyelitis and its prevention is crucial to minimizing the incidence of this dangerous infection. It is important to inform patients about appropriate wound care practices, such as how to properly clean and dress wounds and how urgently to seek medical attention if they exhibit any signs of infection.

Patients who have underlying medical disorders that increase their risk of osteomyelitis should also receive specialized information on how to manage their disease and reduce risk factors. This could involve recommendations for diabetic patients' blood sugar management, foot hygiene procedures, and methods to strengthen the immune system as a whole.

Patients should also be made aware of the significance of following vaccination regimens, particularly if they are at high risk. Healthcare professionals can enable people to take proactive measures in preventing osteomyelitis and maintaining optimal bone health by actively involving patients in their own treatment and giving them the required tools and knowledge.

CHAPTER SIX

DIFFICULTIES AND RISK AREAS

Risk Factors For Osteomyelitis Development

Numerous risk factors can lead to the development of osteomyelitis, a dangerous bone infection. An open wound or other damage that exposes the bone to microorganisms is one of the main causes. Individuals with compromised immune systems, including those with diabetes or HIV/AIDS, are also more vulnerable since their bodies may find it difficult to properly combat infections. Furthermore, illnesses including sickle cell anemia and peripheral vascular disease can reduce blood supply to the bones, increasing their vulnerability to infection.

Recent surgery or the presence of medical equipment like implants or catheters, which can bring bacteria into the body, are important risk factors as well. Osteomyelitis risk is further increased by chronic disorders that impair blood circulation, such as peripheral artery disease or chronic venous insufficiency. These factors decrease the body's capacity to supply immune cells and antibiotics to the infected bone.

In addition, some lifestyle choices—such as smoking or injecting drugs—can impair immunity and make people more vulnerable to illnesses like osteomyelitis. Inadequately treated chronic illnesses, such as diabetes or rheumatoid arthritis, can also hinder the body's natural healing process, making it easier for bacteria to infiltrate the bones.

Determining these risk factors is essential for osteomyelitis early diagnosis and prevention. Professionals in healthcare can lower the risk of infection and enhance patient outcomes by being proactive in identifying the underlying causes.

Possible Difficulties

Numerous consequences from osteomyelitis can have a serious negative effect on a person's quality of life. Chronic pain is one of the most frequent side effects, and it can linger even after the infection has been treated. The infection's inflammation and resulting bone tissue destruction can cause persistent discomfort that hinders movement and interferes with day-to-day activities.

Osteomyelitis can occasionally result in limb malformation, especially if it damages an adult's bone structure or disrupts the growth plates in youngsters. This may lead to cosmetic problems and functional impairment, which could lower someone's confidence and self-esteem. In addition, surgical procedures such as bone debridement or amputation may be necessary in severe cases of osteomyelitis in order to remove contaminated tissue and stop the infection from spreading.

The infection spreading to nearby tissues or the bloodstream, which could result in sepsis and systemic sickness, is another possible consequence. If supportive care and antibiotics are not administered right away, this could become fatal. Recurrent osteomyelitis episodes can also weaken the damaged bone and raise the chance of future fractures or infections.

Addressing these consequences needs a comprehensive approach that involves medical treatment, rehabilitation, and regular monitoring to prevent long-term disability and improve the patient's overall well-being.

Effects On Mobility And Everyday Life

Osteomyelitis can have a significant influence on everyday functioning and mobility, impacting not just physical health but also mental and emotional well-being. Everyday activities, including work, school, and social relationships, can be disrupted by chronic pain, limited mobility, and the need for continuous medical attention.

Osteomyelitis patients may find it difficult to walk or carry out basic duties because of pain, stiffness, and weakness in the affected leg. They may become dependent on others for help with everyday tasks or mobility devices like crutches or wheelchairs, which can cause emotions of frustration, loneliness, and dependency.

Furthermore, the psychological toll of dealing with a chronic illness like osteomyelitis should not be overlooked.

Chronic pain, physical restrictions, and the unknown nature of future consequences can all lead to worry, sadness, and a lower standard of living. In order to promote holistic healing and rehabilitation, healthcare professionals must address not just the physical symptoms of the ailment but also its emotional and social elements.

People can manage the difficulties of having osteomyelitis and enhance their general quality of life by keeping a good outlook, continuing to participate in worthwhile activities, and asking for help from family, friends, and medical experts.

Techniques To Reduce Difficulties

Osteomyelitis consequences must be minimized by a multimodal strategy that takes into account the infection's effects on the surrounding tissues and the damaged bone as well as the underlying cause.

Antibiotics must be used promptly and appropriately to treat acute infections in order to stop the spread of bacteria and lower the risk of consequences like deformity, chronic discomfort, and systemic sickness.

Early intervention can help stop the infection from spreading and reduce bone damage in situations where surgical intervention is required, such as the drainage of abscesses or the removal of infected tissue. Surgical methods like bone grafting and debridement can be used to remove contaminated tissue and encourage the afflicted bone to recover.

It is also possible to lessen the chance of recurring infections and consequences by improving general health and treating underlying risk factors.

This could involve treating long-term illnesses like diabetes or peripheral vascular disease, enhancing wound care procedures, and encouraging healthy lifestyle choices like quitting smoking and getting regular exercise.

To spot and treat any possible issues early on, close observation and follow-up treatment are also essential. Frequent imaging examinations, laboratory testing, and medical evaluations can assist monitor treatment progress, identifying any indications of infection problems or recurrence, and modifying the treatment plan as necessary to maximize results.

Healthcare professionals can lessen the effects of osteomyelitis on patients' lives and enhance their general prognosis and quality of life by putting these measures into practice.

The Value Of Frequently Following Up

For those healing from osteomyelitis, routine follow-up care is crucial in order to track their development, identify any indications of infection recurrence or consequences, and modify their treatment plan as necessary. Follow-up consultations with medical professionals provide continuous assessment of the healing process, evaluation of any lingering symptoms or functional restrictions, and refinement of treatment plans to support sustained recovery.

In order to determine the condition of the damaged bone and surrounding tissues, medical professionals may run laboratory tests, examine imaging studies, and conduct physical examinations during follow-up visits. To avoid more problems, any indications of an infection recurrence, such as continuous discomfort, swelling, or drainage from the wound site, should be assessed and treated very quickly.

Follow-up care may include rehabilitation therapies like physical therapy or occupational therapy in addition to medical examination in order to restore function, strength, and mobility to the damaged limb. `

These treatments can lessen the chance of long-term disability, help people regain their independence, and enhance their quality of life.

In addition, follow-up visits give medical professionals a chance to answer any queries or concerns patients may have regarding their illness, course of treatment, or recuperation period. It is imperative that patients and healthcare providers engage in transparent communication and teamwork to guarantee that patients receive the necessary support and assistance to effectively manage the challenges of living with osteomyelitis and attain optimal outcomes.

Healthcare professionals can empower people healing from osteomyelitis to actively participate in their own health and well-being and foster long-term success in managing their illness by highlighting the significance of routine follow-up care.

CHAPTER SEVEN

ORTHOPAEDIC OSTEOMYELIA

Particular Difficulties In Pediatric Cases

Osteomyelitis in children presents special issues due to their developing skeletal structures and immune systems. The difficulty of promptly detecting the disease is one major obstacle. Children's symptoms may not always be evident to them, and symptoms like fever and localized pain can indicate a number of different ailments. Furthermore, it can be challenging to differentiate between osteomyelitis and common childhood injuries in children because they are generally active and may sustain minor injuries regularly.

Furthermore, compared to adult osteomyelitis, pediatric osteomyelitis can present with different symptoms. In cases involving children, symptoms might not be as noticeable at first, delaying identification and treatment.

Delays like these raise the possibility of consequences like joint issues or malformations of the bones.

In addition, since children's bones are still developing, osteomyelitis may disrupt bone growth and could cause long-term problems.

Children's Diagnosis And Treatment Considerations

In addition to other diagnostic tests, a comprehensive clinical evaluation is necessary for the diagnosis of osteomyelitis in children. Healthcare professionals must rely on a mix of physical examinations, imaging studies like X-rays or MRI scans, and laboratory testing like blood cultures to confirm the diagnosis because children may not always be able to convey their symptoms clearly.

A bone biopsy might be required in some circumstances in order to determine the causing organism.

Antibiotics and, occasionally, surgery are used in combination for treatment when a diagnosis has been made.

In order to guarantee optimal delivery of antibiotics, intravenous administration is utilized, particularly in situations when the infection has deeply permeated the bone.

The presumed organism's sensitivity to various drugs determines which antibiotics are best. In cases where conservative treatment is ineffective or there is a risk of bone necrosis, surgery may be necessary to drain abscesses or remove contaminated tissue.

Long-Term Impacts on Development and Growth

Childhood growth and development can be significantly impacted by osteomyelitis over an extended period of time. Since the infection affects the bone, it may cause anomalies in the development of the skeleton by interfering with bone growth. Severe cases may lead to abnormalities in the joints or variations in the length of the limbs, which can affect movement and function.

Furthermore, long-term antibiotic usage can upset the usual balance of intestinal flora and could have an impact on nutritional absorption, particularly during crucial growth stages. Children's general growth and development may be further impacted by this.

Furthermore, children's quality of life and emotional well-being may be negatively impacted psychologically by osteomyelitis-related chronic pain or functional limitations.

Effects Of Psychology On Families And Children

The diagnosis and treatment of osteomyelitis can take a toll on children and their families both emotionally and psychologically.

Due to the pain and discomfort of the ailment, as well as the disruption it brings to their regular routines and activities, children may experience fear, anxiety, or dissatisfaction. If they need lengthy medical care or have physical restrictions, they could also feel alone or unlike their peers.

Handling a child's illness can be emotionally taxing for families. Parents may feel overwhelmed by the demands of managing their child's care, organizing medical visits, and navigating the healthcare system. They may also have emotions of shame or self-blame, wondering if they could have done anything to prevent the infection. Healthcare professionals must provide children and their families with resources and assistance in order to help them deal with the psychological effects of osteomyelitis.

Prevention Techniques Particular To Pediatrics

A comprehensive strategy that takes into account both general risk factors and pediatric-specific ones is needed to prevent osteomyelitis in children.

In order to lower the risk of bacterial infections, one essential component is encouraging basic hygiene practices, such as frequent handwashing and appropriate wound care. In order to safeguard their children against common diseases that might cause osteomyelitis, parents should also make sure that their children obtain routine vaccines.

Furthermore, any wounds or infections that could raise the risk of osteomyelitis must be treated right away.

This entails appropriately cleaning and bandaging wounds as well as obtaining medical help if infection symptoms appear.

Close observation and preventive actions are especially crucial for kids with underlying medical disorders like diabetes or sickle cell disease that may compromise their immune systems.

Providing early detection and treatment with education to children and their families regarding the symptoms and indicators of osteomyelitis might also be beneficial. Providing options for obtaining medical attention and promoting open communication can enable families to take charge of their children's health.

Healthcare professionals can lessen the effects of this potentially dangerous illness and help lower the occurrence of osteomyelitis in juvenile populations by putting these preventative methods into practice.

CHAPTER EIGHT

MANAGING OSTEOMYELITIS

Changes In Lifestyle

Living with osteomyelitis frequently necessitates considerable adjustments to routines and habits.

Changing to a healthy lifestyle can help with symptom management and general health enhancement.

First and foremost, bone health depends on eating a balanced diet full of vital elements like calcium and vitamin D. Including foods that are high in nutrients, such as fish, dairy products, and leafy greens, can help strengthen and repair bones.

It's crucial to give up bad habits like smoking and binge drinking that might make the illness worse.

The body may find it more difficult to fight infections and heal from osteomyelitis as a result of these drugs' potential to affect blood circulation and bone health.

Both drinking enough water and getting enough sleep are critical for boosting the body's immune system.

Exercise on a regular basis that is adapted to your individual needs and capabilities is crucial. Walking, swimming, and cycling are examples of low-impact exercises that can enhance circulation and accelerate healing without placing undue strain on the bones. When beginning a new exercise program, always check with your doctor to make sure it's safe and appropriate for your condition.

Exercises For Rehabilitation

Exercises for rehabilitation are essential to osteomyelitis recovery and strength and mobility restoration.

To make sure these exercises are appropriate for your condition and growth, a physical therapist usually designs and oversees their execution.

Exercises that improve range of motion are frequently the first step in recovery. The flexibility of the muscles and joints surrounding the injured area is preserved and enhanced by these workouts.

Stiffness can be avoided and general function can be enhanced with mild stretching and mobility activities.

The next round of exercises involves strengthening, with an emphasis on developing the muscles that support the injured bones. Without overstretching their bones, patients can gradually regain strength with bodyweight exercises, resistance bands, or modest weights.

Additionally, it is crucial to strengthen your core since it promotes good body mechanics and lowers your chance of sustaining new injuries.

Exercises for balance and coordination are included to increase stability and reduce the risk of falls, which can be especially dangerous for someone with weak bones. Proprioception and general balance can be enhanced by exercises like one-leg stands and balance boards.

Coping Mechanisms And Emotional Assistance

Having a long-term illness such as osteomyelitis can be emotionally taxing. It's critical to have strong coping mechanisms and a support network in place. A sense of understanding and belonging can be obtained through emotional support from friends, family, and support groups. This is important for mental health.

For the purpose of treating the psychological effects of having a chronic illness, counseling or therapy may be helpful. The development of coping mechanisms to manage osteomyelitis-related pain, anxiety, and depression is a specialty of cognitive-behavioral therapy (CBT).

Stress can be decreased and general mental health can be enhanced by practicing relaxation techniques such as progressive muscle relaxation, deep breathing, and mindfulness meditation. A mental vacation from the day-to-day difficulties of controlling osteomyelitis can also be obtained through interests and pursuits that make you happy and feel accomplished.

Extended-Term Management Strategies

Osteomyelitis requires a multifaceted approach for long-term management, including medication, dietary modifications, and routine monitoring. Following the recommended antibiotic regimen is essential to guaranteeing that the illness is fully treated.

It's essential to schedule follow-up visits with medical professionals on a regular basis to assess progress and modify the treatment plan as needed.

Continuing to live a healthy lifestyle is an essential component of long-term care. A balanced diet, consistent exercise, and abstaining from bad habits are all part of this. Keeping the lines of communication open with your medical professionals guarantees that any new symptoms or issues are taken care of right away.

In order to stop reinfection, self-care procedures are crucial. These include wound care for surgical sites and open sores. Additionally, patients need to be on the lookout for any recurrence symptoms, such as increasing pain, swelling, or redness in the vicinity of the affected area.

Keeping An Eye Out For Recurrence

Because osteomyelitis tends to reoccur, close observation is essential.

Frequent medical check-ups, which include imaging investigations and blood testing, aid in the early detection of any recurrence signals. Any new or worsening symptoms, such as persistent pain, fever, or changes in the affected area's condition, should be reported by the patient.

Recurrence risk can be considerably decreased by being aware of possible symptoms and taking a proactive approach to medical care.

Establishing a regular self-monitoring regimen and seeking professional medical supervision together guarantee that any recurrence is identified early and treated quickly, reducing problems and enhancing long-term health.

CHAPTER NINE

SCIENCE AND UPCOMING VIEWS

Current Research Trends In Osteomyelitis

New discoveries in the field of osteomyelitis research are opening doors to improved methods of diagnosis, care, and prevention. The growing use of genetic and molecular methods to comprehend the pathophysiology of osteomyelitis is one noteworthy trend.

Genome sequencing is being used by researchers to pinpoint the precise bacterial strains causing infections and to comprehend the mechanisms underlying their resistance. This genetic knowledge is essential for creating individualized treatment regimens and focused antibiotics.

The investigation of biofilm dynamics in osteomyelitis is another noteworthy development.

The persistent nature of the illness is mostly due to biofilms, which are intricate populations of bacteria that stick to surfaces. Researchers can better understand how bacteria elude the immune system and fight antibiotics to cause persistent illnesses by studying biofilms. The development of novel treatments targeted at preventing biofilm formation and boosting the effectiveness of antibiotics is being guided by this research.

Treatment Strategies That Look Good

Novel therapeutic modalities for osteomyelitis are very promising. The application of antimicrobial peptides is among the most intriguing developments (AMPs). Compared to conventional antibiotics, these naturally occurring compounds are less likely to cause resistance and are capable of eliminating a broad variety of bacteria.

By improving their stability and efficacy, AMPs can be designed to be a potent new weapon in the fight against osteomyelitis.

Furthermore, more efficient medication delivery methods are being developed by utilizing the latest developments in nanotechnology. Antibiotics can be specifically formulated into nanoparticles that are delivered to the infection site, increasing local medication concentrations and minimizing systemic side effects. This focused strategy reduces the likelihood of antibiotic resistance while simultaneously increasing therapeutic efficacy.

Osteomyelitis treatment is also progressing thanks to regenerative medicine. To encourage bone healing and regeneration in patients with osteomyelitis, methods like bone grafting, tissue engineering, and the use of stem cells are being improved. The goal of these techniques is to repair the integrity and function of bones, which are frequently damaged by persistent infections.

Obstacles In Prevention And Treatment

Notwithstanding these developments, treating and preventing osteomyelitis still presents a number of difficulties.

The challenge of correctly and early diagnosis of the disease is one of the main obstacles. A precise diagnosis of osteomyelitis frequently necessitates a combination of imaging scans, microbiological tests, and clinical assessment because the condition can mirror other conditions. This intricacy has the potential to worsen therapy effects by delaying it.

The emergence of germs resistant to antibiotics is another problem. Antibiotic-resistant organisms have emerged as a result of overuse and abuse of antibiotics, making infections more difficult to treat. To keep ahead of resistant bacteria, new antibiotics and alternative medicines must be continuously developed.

Osteomyelitis prevention is still a major concern, particularly in high-risk populations like diabetics and people with orthopedic implants.

Enhancing wound care, hygienic habits, and early intervention for persons who are at risk are crucial strategies that necessitate ongoing education and funding.

The Value Of Multidisciplinary Cooperation

The complexity of osteomyelitis necessitates a multidisciplinary team effort to address. Collaboration among infectious disease experts, orthopedic surgeons, microbiologists, and bioengineers is necessary to create complete treatment plans and creative fixes. Innovations in single disciplines may not catch up with interdisciplinary research; an example of this is the fusion of fresh therapeutic methods with state-of-the-art imaging tools.

Furthermore, cooperation involves researchers and medical professionals working together to apply lab results to clinical settings. This guarantees that patients receive the most recent developments in osteomyelitis care and therapy.

Promoting And Endorsing Osteomyelitis Research

To further osteomyelitis research, advocacy, and support are crucial. Expanded financial support from both public and private entities can quicken research endeavors and enable extensive clinical studies. In order to encourage early detection and intervention, public awareness initiatives can also be extremely important in educating the public about the dangers and symptoms of osteomyelitis.

Networks of support are just as crucial for osteomyelitis patients and their families. These networks help people deal with the difficulties brought on by the illness by offering helpful resources, consoling, and useful guidance. In order to maintain osteomyelitis research as a top priority on the medical research agenda, advocacy groups can also have an impact on policy decisions.

Even though osteomyelitis research is making great progress, more innovation, cooperation, and support are needed to enhance patient outcomes globally due to enduring difficulties.

www.ingramcontent.com/pod-product-compliance
Lightning Source LLC
Chambersburg PA
CBHW071841210526
45479CB00001B/228